The Art
of
Aromatherapy

An Expert's Guide to Using Essential Oils for Health and Well-Being

By

Dr. Justin D. Morales

Disclaimer

Content

Introduction

Being a young boy, I always had a fascination with plants and nature. I loved spending time outdoors, studying the different types of plants and their unique properties. As I grew older, I became interested in the art of aromatherapy and the healing powers of essential oils. I was determined to learn everything I could about essential oils and how they could be used to promote health and well-being. I read books, attended workshops, and even enrolled in a course to become a certified aromatherapist.

After completing my training, I decided to open my own aromatherapy practice. I carefully curated a selection of essential oils and created custom blends to help my clients with a variety of health concerns.

On a particular day, a woman named Claire came to my practice seeking help for her chronic migraines. She had tried many different treatments, but nothing seemed to provide lasting relief. I listened carefully as she described her symptoms and lifestyle. I then recommended a custom blend of essential oils, including lavender, peppermint, and eucalyptus, to be used for inhalation and topical application. She was skeptical at first, but she was willing to try anything to find relief from her migraines. She followed my instructions and began using the essential oil blend regularly. She was surprised, as she began to experience relief from her migraines. The scent of the oils provided a calming effect, and the anti-inflammatory properties helped to reduce the intensity of her headaches. As time went by, Claire's migraines became less frequent and less severe. She was astonished at the power of essential oils and grateful for my expertise and guidance. I was proud of the impact I was making on people's lives and felt grateful to be able to share my knowledge and passion for the art of aromatherapy.

For millennia, essential oils have been utilized for their medicinal and healing powers. These oils are derived from plants, flowers, and herbs and contain potent components that are beneficial to both the body and the mind. Aromatherapy is the practice of using essential oils to enhance health and well-being. It has grown in popularity in recent years as people seek natural and holistic methods to wellbeing.

In "The Art of Aromatherapy: An Expert's Guide to Using Essential Oils for Health and Well-Being," we will dig into the intriguing realm of aromatherapy and the numerous ways essential oils may enhance physical, emotional, and mental health. Whether you're new to essential oils or a seasoned practitioner, this book will equip you with the information and skills you need to harness nature's power and attain maximum well-being.

This book will teach you how essential oils work, how to select the best oils for your requirements, and how to use them safely and successfully. We will discuss essential oils for physical health, mental well-being, beauty and self-care, and house and environment. You'll also discover helpful hints, recipes, and instructions for making your own unique mixes to treat specific health conditions. This book is based on a genuine appreciation for the power and potential of essential oils. We think that when used with thought and care, these oils may help us live more balanced and fulfilled lives. Whether you want to treat a specific health issue or just improve your general well-being, "The Art of Aromatherapy" will provide you the knowledge and motivation you need to take control of your health and embrace the healing power of essential oils.

Chapter 1

Understanding Essential Oils

Essential oils are highly volatile liquids derived from plants, flowers, and herbs. These oils include the concentrated essence of the plant as well as a number of potent chemicals like terpenes, esters, aldehydes, ketones, and phenols. Each essential oil has its own chemical composition, which gives it a particular scent and set of qualities.

In this chapter, we'll go over the fundamentals of essential oils, such as how they're extracted, how they operate, and how to select high-quality oils.

Methods of Extraction

Steam distillation, cold pressing, and solvent extraction are all processes for extracting essential oils from plants. The most popular process is steam distillation, which involves heating the plant material to extract the essential oil. Cold pressing is a method of extracting citrus oils that includes pressing the fruit to release the oil. Solvent extraction involves extracting the oil using a solvent and is utilized for fragile plant materials such as flowers.

Composition of Chemicals

Essential oils are a complex blend of chemicals, each with its own set of qualities. Terpenes, esters, aldehydes, ketones, and phenols are some of the most prevalent chemical families found in essential oils. Essential oils are a diverse and effective tool for health and wellness since each chemical family has a different effect on the body and mind.

How Essential Oils Function

Through the sense of smell and physical application, essential oils interact with the chemistry of the body. When essential oils are breathed, their molecules go down the nasal passages and into the limbic system, which is the area of the brain responsible for emotions, memory, and behavior. This can have a significant impact on one's mood and mental well-being.

When essential oils are used topically, they can permeate the skin and reach the circulation, where they can have a systemic influence on the body. This is why it is critical to use high-quality oils that are free of impurities and properly diluted to avoid skin irritation.

Selecting High-Quality Oils

Because not all essential oils are made equal, it is critical to select high-quality oils that are pure, powerful, and free of impurities. Look for oils labeled "pure" or "therapeutic grade" and obtained from reliable firms that adhere to sustainable and ethical practices. Oils labeled "fragrance oils" or "perfume oils" should be avoided since they may include synthetic components and additions.

To summarize, knowing essential oils is critical for utilizing them safely and successfully. You may make educated decisions regarding oils and how to use them to support your health and well-being by knowing about their extraction processes, chemical makeup, and how they perform. The next chapter will go through some of the most common essential oils and their attributes.

Chapter 2

Using Essential Oils Safely

While essential oils provide a variety of health and wellness advantages, it is critical to utilize them cautiously to avoid unwanted reactions. In this chapter, we will look at the fundamentals of essential oil safety, such as dilution, topical administration, and inhalation.

Dilution

To minimize skin irritation and other negative responses, essential oils should always be diluted before usage. A little amount of essential oil is diluted with a carrier oil, such as coconut or jojoba oil. The proportion of essential oil to carrier oil will vary depending on the oil and the intended usage, but a 2% dilution is a fair rule of thumb for most uses.

Application Topically

It is critical to apply essential oils correctly to avoid skin irritation and sensitization when using them topically. Always do a patch test by applying a tiny amount of diluted oil to a small area of skin and waiting 24 hours to see if there are any negative responses. Applying oils to sensitive regions such as the eyes, nose, or genitals is not recommended.

Inhalation

Another typical application for essential oils is inhalation, but exercise caution to avoid overexposure. Essential oils should never be inhaled directly from the bottle or for a lengthy period of time. Diffuse oils in a well-ventilated space instead, and restrict inhalation to 15-30 minutes at a time.

Additional Safety Considerations

Other safety precautions to bear in mind while utilizing essential oils include dilution, topical use, and inhalation. These are some examples:
Keep essential oils away from children and pets.
Do not consume essential oils unless you are under the supervision of a certified healthcare practitioner.

If you are pregnant or nursing, have a medical condition, or are on medication, avoid using essential oils.

Keep essential oils cold and dark, away from sunshine and heat.

By adhering to these essential oil safety guidelines, you may reap the numerous advantages of these potent oils without jeopardizing your health.

Conclusion

It is critical to use essential oils carefully in order to realize their advantages and avoid unwanted effects. Dilution, topical use, and inhalation are all significant concerns, as are other safety precautions like keeping oils out of the reach of children and pets and properly storing them. You may use the power of nature to enhance your health and well-being by utilizing essential oils wisely and safely.

Chapter 3

Essential Oils for Physical Health

For decades, essential oils have been utilized to enhance physical health, from curing minor diseases to boosting general wellness. We will look at some of the most popular essential oils for physical health and their qualities in this chapter.

Peppermint Oil

Peppermint oil is well-known for its refreshing and energizing effects. It may be used topically to relieve muscular pain and headaches, as well as respiratory disorders like congestion and coughing. Peppermint oil can also be used to treat digestive problems such as bloating, nausea, and indigestion.

Lavender Essential Oil

Lavender oil is a versatile oil that is widely used for stress treatment and relaxation. It also aids in the promotion of peaceful sleep and can be used topically to treat minor skin irritations such as bug bites and burns. Lavender oil also has antibacterial qualities and may be used to treat small wounds and scrapes.

Tea Tree Essential Oil

Tea tree oil is a potent antiseptic that may be used to treat a variety of skin conditions such as acne, eczema, and fungal infections. It may also be used as a natural insect repellent and is beneficial for respiratory ailments such as coughing and congestion.

Eucalyptus Oil

Because it helps to remove congestion and encourage better breathing, eucalyptus oil is often used for respiratory disorders such as colds and flu. It is also an effective insect repellent and may be used topically to relieve mild muscular and joint discomfort.

Frankincense Oil

Because of its relaxing and centering characteristics, frankincense oil is a popular choice for meditation and relaxation. It can also be used topically to minimize the appearance of fine lines and wrinkles and to promote healthy skin.

Other Physical Health Essential Oils

There are numerous additional oils that may be utilized to enhance physical health in addition to the essential oils described above. Some examples are:
Lemon oil, which may be utilized as a natural detoxifier and can aid with digestion.
Rosemary oil is widely used to promote hair development and reduce hair loss.
Chamomile oil can relieve skin irritation and promote deep sleep.

Conclusion

Essential oils may be a very effective tool for promoting physical health and wellness. Some of the various oils that may be utilized for a variety of physical health conditions are peppermint oil, lavender oil, tea tree oil, eucalyptus oil, and frankincense oil. It is critical to follow safe usage recommendations when using essential oils for physical health and to check with a certified healthcare practitioner if you have any medical issues or are taking medication. The advantages of essential oils for emotional and mental well-being will be discussed in the next chapter.

Chapter 4

Essential Oils for Emotional Well-Being

For millennia, essential oils have been utilized to promote emotional well-being. We will look at the advantages of essential oils for mental health and some of the most popular oils for this purpose in this chapter.

Lemon Juice

Lemon oil is well-known for its energizing and uplifting effects. It can assist to boost one's mood as well as lessen tension and anxiety. Lemon oil can also help with attention and concentration.

Lavender Essential Oil

Lavender oil is a versatile oil that is widely used for stress treatment and relaxation. It can assist to alleviate anxiety and produce sensations of peace and relaxation. Lavender oil can also aid in the promotion of peaceful sleep and the reduction of irritation.

Ylang Ylang Essential Oil

Ylang Ylang oil is a flower oil with relaxing and soothing characteristics. It can assist to alleviate tension and anxiety while also promoting relaxation and tranquility. Aphrodisiac properties are also associated with Ylang Ylang oil.

Bergamot Essential Oil

Bergamot oil is a citrus oil that is often used for its mood-lifting and elevating effects. It can assist to alleviate anxiety and sadness while increasing emotions of pleasure and well-being. Bergamot oil can also aid in the reduction of weariness and the improvement of mental clarity.

Frankincense Oil

Because of its relaxing and centering characteristics, frankincense oil is a popular choice for meditation and relaxation. It can aid in the reduction of worry and the promotion of inner calm and tranquility. Frankincense oil can also aid in the reduction of irritation and the promotion of emotional equilibrium.

Other Emotional Well-Being Essential Oils

There are many additional oils that may be used to improve mental well-being in addition to the essential oils described above. Some examples are:

Chamomile oil, which can assist to alleviate anxiety while also promoting sensations of tranquility and relaxation.
Patchouli oil, which is frequently used to boost self-confidence and inner strength.
Rose oil can assist to alleviate stress and increase emotions of contentment and well-being.

Conclusion

Essential oils may be a very effective technique for enhancing emotional well-being. Some of the various oils that may be utilized for mental wellness are lemon oil, lavender oil, ylang ylang oil, bergamot oil, and frankincense oil. It is critical to follow safe usage recommendations when using essential oils for emotional well-being and to speak with a trained healthcare practitioner if you have any medical issues or are taking medication.

Chapter 5

Essential Oils for Beauty and Self-Care

Essential oils may be a very effective complement to any beauty or self-care regimen. In this chapter, we'll look at the advantages of essential oils for beauty and self-care, as well as some of the more popular ones.

Tea Tree Essential Oil

Because of its antibacterial and antifungal characteristics, tea tree oil is a popular essential oil for skin care. It can aid in the treatment of acne, the reduction of inflammation, and the general look of the skin. Tea tree oil is also effective in treating dandruff and other scalp disorders.

Lavender Essential Oil

Lavender oil is a versatile oil that is widely used for stress treatment and relaxation. It may also be used for skin care by soothing and healing irritated or inflamed skin. Lavender oil can also aid in the promotion of peaceful sleep, the reduction of anxiety, and the improvement of mood.

Frankincense Oil

Frankincense oil is a well-known anti-aging and skin regeneration oil. It can aid in the reduction of fine lines and wrinkles, the improvement of skin suppleness, and the promotion of general skin health. Frankincense oil may also be used to relax and relieve tension.

Rosehip Seed Oil

Rosehip oil is a popular skin care oil because it is high in antioxidants and necessary fatty acids. It can aid in the improvement of skin texture and tone, the reduction of scars and fine lines, and the promotion of general skin health. Rosehip oil is also useful for moisturising and nourishing dry or sensitive skin.

Peppermint Oil

Peppermint oil is a revitalising oil that may be used to care for your hair. It can aid in the improvement of scalp health, the reduction of dandruff, and the promotion of hair growth. Peppermint oil can also help with headaches and enhance mental clarity.

Other Beauty and Self-Care Essential Oils

There are numerous additional oils that may be used for beauty and self-care in addition to the essential oils described above. Some examples are:

Geranium oil, which can assist to balance natural oil production in the skin and promote healthy skin.
Lemon oil can assist to brighten and tone the skin while also reducing the appearance of age spots and discolouration.
Chamomile oil has the ability to soothe and repair inflamed skin while also promoting general skin health.

Conclusion

Essential oils may be an extremely beneficial addition to any beauty or self-care regimen. Some of the various oils that may be used for beauty and self-care are tea tree oil, lavender oil, frankincense oil, rosehip oil, and peppermint oil. It is critical to follow safe usage recommendations when using essential oils for skin or hair care, and to contact with a skilled healthcare practitioner if you have any medical issues or are taking medication. The benefits of essential oils for cleaning and home usage will be discussed in the next chapter.

Chapter 6

Essential Oils for Home and Environment

Natural alternatives to chemical-laden cleaning products and air fresheners include essential oils. In this chapter, we'll look at the advantages of utilising essential oils for cleaning and domestic usage, as well as some of the most popular oils for the job.

Lemon Juice

Lemon oil is a multipurpose oil that is frequently used for cleaning and disinfecting. It can aid in the removal of oil and dirt from surfaces, as well as the elimination of germs and viruses. Lemon oil may also be used to refresh the air and lift one's spirits.

Tea Tree Essential Oil

Tea tree oil is another effective cleaning and disinfecting oil. It may aid in the removal of mold, mildew, and other microorganisms, making it an excellent choice for usage in bathrooms and kitchens. Tea tree oil may also be used to promote respiratory health and refresh the air.

Eucalyptus Oil

Eucalyptus oil is a revitalising oil that is frequently used for cleaning and disinfecting. It can aid in the removal of odours and microorganisms while also improving respiratory health. Insect and pest repellents can also be made from eucalyptus oil.

Peppermint Oil

Peppermint oil is a revitalising oil that is frequently used in cleaning and disinfecting. It can assist to remove odours and germs while also repelling insects and pests. Peppermint oil can also help with mental clarity and attention.

Other Home and Environment Essential Oils

Aside from the essential oils listed above, there are other additional oils that may be utilised for cleaning and domestic purposes. Some examples are:

Lavender oil may be used to refresh the air while also improving relaxation and sleep.
Grapefruit oil, which may be used to eradicate smells and boost mood.
Rosemary oil may be used to repel insects and vermin as well as to increase mental clarity.

Conclusion

Essential oils may be an excellent complement to any cleaning or air-freshening regimen. Lemon oil, tea tree oil, eucalyptus oil, and peppermint oil are just a few examples of oils that may be utilised for cleaning and domestic purposes. It is critical to follow safe usage standards and utilise adequate dilution when using essential oils for cleaning.

Conclusion

We've looked at the huge realm of aromatherapy and the various ways essential oils may be used to enhance health and well-being throughout this book. We've studied about the history of aromatherapy as well as the science behind how essential oils may help our physical and mental wellbeing.

We've looked at essential oil safety requirements and the many various ways they may be utilized, including as for physical health, mental well-being, beauty and self-care, and home and environment. We learned about the many essential oils and their distinct qualities and advantages.

One of the most important things to remember while utilising essential oils is to do it safely and correctly. Essential oils are highly concentrated compounds that must be handled with caution. Always dilute oils properly and avoid using oils that might cause irritation or allergic responses.

It is also crucial to remember that, while essential oils have several advantages, they should not be taken in place of medical therapy. If you have major health issues, you should contact with a healthcare practitioner before taking essential oils.

Aromatherapy is an excellent approach to improve our physical and mental health, as well as our general well-being. We can enjoy a range of advantages by introducing essential oils into our everyday routines, including improved mood, better sleep, higher energy, and enhanced immunological function.

I hope this book has given you the knowledge and skills you need to start using essential oils in your own life. Always use them cautiously and correctly

to get the numerous benefits that aromatherapy has
to offer.